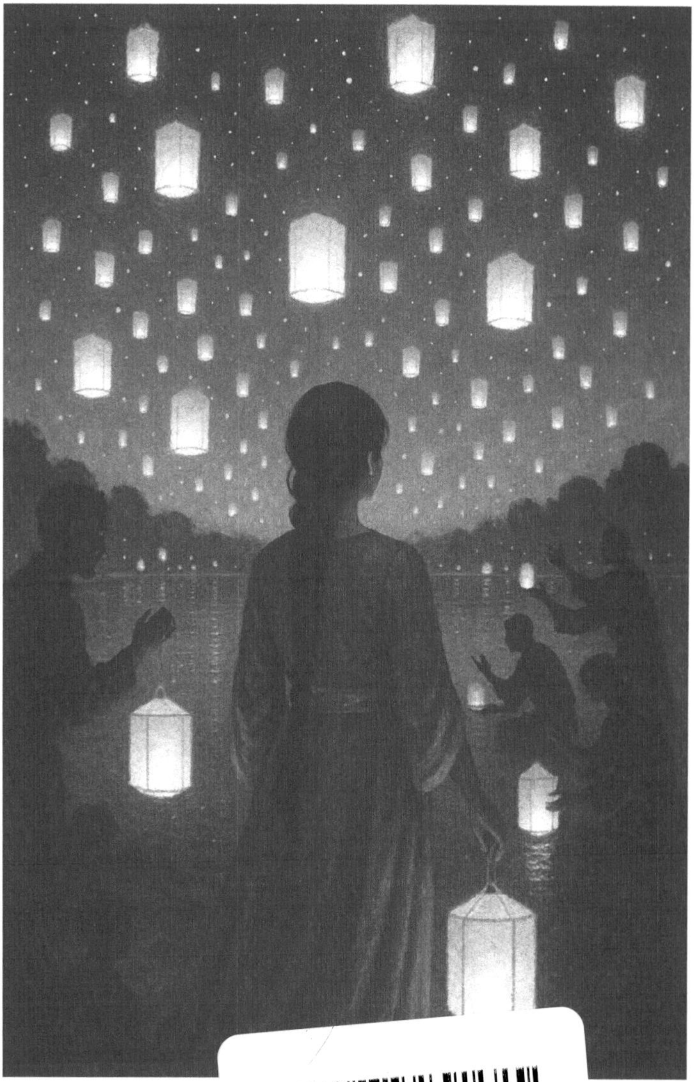

AF516924

First Published by Ink Gladiators Press®
Copyright © 2025 Reena Doss
Translations Of Hope

Editor-in-Chief: Reena Doss

First Edition
ISBN 13: 978-93-49117-48-8

Self-Boundaries For You - Lantern 8

Credits:

Book Design by Leonie Belle Hawk
Turkish & Swahili Translations: Edited and Proofed by Justin Adam Wolf and Aelius Arche

All rights reserved. This edition may only be distributed by the author and publisher. The contents of this book are the author's perceptions, observations, and insights, based on her individual experiences. Any resemblance to real persons is unintended and should not be inferred. The moral rights of the author and publisher have been asserted. No part of this book may be reproduced in any form, or by electronic, AI or mechanical means, including information storage and retrieval systems, without written permission from the author, with the only exception being made for a reviewer who may quote brief passages in a review.

Disclaimer: The views and opinions expressed by the author are personal and do not represent those of Ink Gladiators Press®, its staff, communities, or affiliates, unless explicitly stated.

Ink Gladiators Press®
Publishing and promoting warriors on life's battlefield
Founded in 2019 | Bangalore, India
www.inkgladiatorspress.com

To my beloved Weaver,

Thank you for making each of us so unique,
with our own history, experiences and choices;
may we always use the gift of free will to serve you
in every possible way with all that we are

To my future family,

may we always search for answers to the big questions,
cherish what we discover individually and together
and uphold our boundaries on what matters the most

To my dear Seekers of Peace,

may you define your affirmations to keep your soul alive
by standing firm on the parts of you that yearn
for what you cultivate on the path ahead

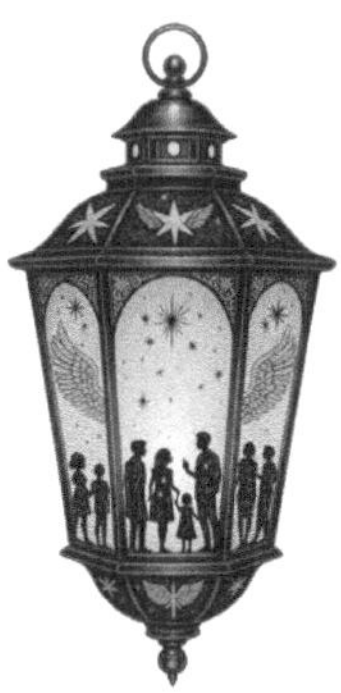

This book is a lantern of

Self-Boundaries For You

Love Adores
Never-ending Tales:
Eagerly Ready, News Sails

Boundaries are a personal checklist that we often have but don't know how to apply and hold them together. Originally written in English, these seeds of thought have been translated into Turkish and Swahili.

SELF BOUNDARIES FOR YOU

Because Mental Health Matters

I stopped numbering my pages because my story is still being written.

Besides, I do like its symbol a lot—a sleeping 8.

I'll find you in the dark because I'm the girl

who loves to stay *lost* amongst the midnight stars

caught up with moonbeams *in a lantern*

trying to find my way back *home*

LANTERNS

The pleasure of watching light move across the night sky against its deep purples, blues and greys is an incredible sight to behold.

Though I have never seen it in person myself except on TV, reels or videos, I would imagine that it mimics the feeling of a thousand golden suns glimmering brighter than the stars behind them. I would imagine that it would capture the feeling of remembering that we are each important because no matter how small or big we are light travels faster than sound. I would imagine it would make anyone who sees them smile, open their hearts as hope flutters like birdsong near their door, and the taste of something indescribably good wraps them warmly.

Lanterns are necessary because igniting hope is the best cure in support of mental health awareness. Many live in darkness, in a state of feeling disillusioned by those they put their faith in and have forgotten how to see their own hearts through eyes that love, but a lantern is meant for just this purpose—to relight someone's candle with kindness, to hold a hand steadily in their shadows, and to listen gently to the broken pieces in others speaking. Sometimes, the truth is simple.

That delicate point between human nature and the desire to do what is good is where we will meet the Author of Love. Love can only be known from the One who created us and even when people (who follow God) make us feel like He isn't real or there for us, one of the best ways to reconnect with Him directly is to love with all your heart—and to balance it with healthy discernment, boundaries and truth in situations where your broken parts might want to do, feel or say the exact opposite. *E.g.: Jesus Christ*

It is my joy to let go of this lantern—as all lanterns must be—for others to find because I want to share something beautiful that I gained and that is mine to offer: You are deeply loved by Heavenly Hands that have constructed, created and command time, space, and distance.

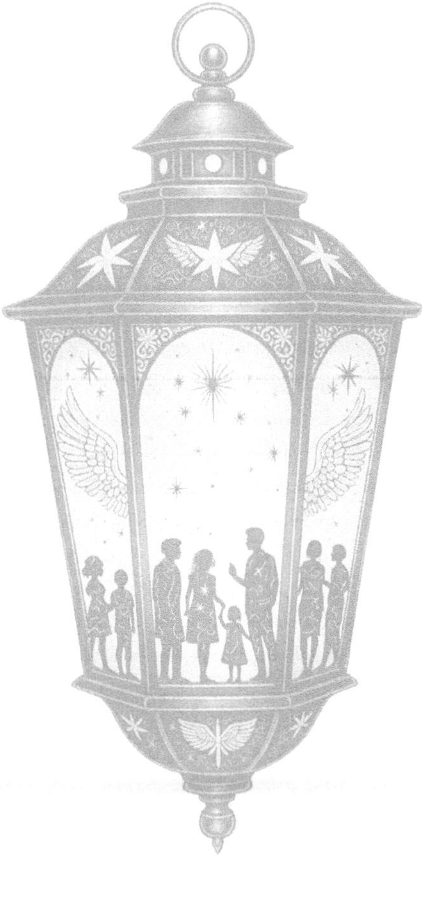

Spiritual Boundaries

"I am my beloved's, and my beloved is mine"

- Song of Solomon 6 : 3

My spiritual affirmations protect my relationship with the Holy Trinity because it keeps my soul committed to trusting that anything in this life is worth it if at the end of it, I get to be with Him who loves me best. This deep connection to my personal faith allows me to respect another person's without needing to override my beliefs or theirs.

In maintaining these boundaries, I might lose those who will misunderstand on purpose because they have unhealed wounds on the subject of religion. I might be seen as not respecting another's faith for being faithful to mine. But as long as I do not condemn, compare, or speak cruelly about another religion, I know that I am being true to myself as well as standing by others. I am okay with being falsely accused as my actions—creative work, words and art reveal more about my nature, even when they don't know why my heart puts the Weaver first, even when it is hard.

I don't stop talking, singing or witnessing the joy of the Lord in my life. I choose Love, because I am made with Love by Love Himself, for Love. How He uses me to give to those who need it the most will always be in the most beautiful way because it will let others know why the Weaver is who He is, not anyone else.

Your spiritual boundaries will be yours.
For me, they are the most important part of me.

What are yours?

Manevi Sınırlar

"Ben sevgilimininim, sevgilim de benimdir."

- Süleyman'ın Şarkısı 6:3

Manevi inançlarım, Kutsal Üçlü ile olan ilişkimi korur, çünkü ruhumun, bu hayattaki her şeyin, sonunda beni en çok seven O'nunla birlikte olacaksam, buna değer olduğuna inanmasını sağlar. Kişisel inancımla olan bu derin bağ, benim ya da başkalarının inançlarını hiçe saymadan, başkalarının inançlarına saygı duymamı sağlar.

Bu sınırları korurken, din konusunda iyileşmemiş yaraları olduğu için kasıtlı olarak yanlış anlayacak olanları kaybedebilirim. Kendi inancıma sadık olduğum için başkalarının inancına saygı duymadığım düşünülebilir. Ancak, başka bir dini kınamadığım, karşılaştırmadığım veya acımasızca konuşmadığım sürece, kendime karşı dürüst olduğumu ve başkalarının yanında olduğumu biliyorum. Yanlış bir şekilde suçlanmayı sorun etmiyorum, çünkü eylemlerim, yaratıcı çalışmalarım, sözlerim ve sanatım, kalbimin neden Weaver'ı her zaman ilk sıraya koyduğunu bilmeseler bile, zor olsa bile, benim doğamı daha iyi ortaya koyuyor.

Hayatımda Rab'bin sevincini konuşmaktan, şarkı söylemekten veya tanıklık etmekten vazgeçmiyorum. Sevgiyi seçiyorum, çünkü ben Sevgi tarafından, Sevgi için, Sevgi ile yaratıldım. O'nun beni en çok ihtiyacı olanlara vermek için kullanması her zaman en güzel şekilde olacaktır, çünkü bu, diğerlerine Weaver'ın neden O olduğunu, başka biri olmadığını gösterecektir.

Ruhsal sınırlarınız size ait olacaktır.
Benim için bunlar benim en önemli parçamdır.

Sizinkiler nelerdir?

Mipaka ya Kiroho

"Mimi ni wa mpenzi wangu, na mpenzi wangu ni wangu"

- Wimbo Ulio Bora 6:3

Thibitisho zangu za kiroho hulinda uhusiano wangu na Utatu Mtakatifu kwa sababu huweka roho yangu imejitolea kuamini kwamba chochote katika maisha haya kina thamani ikiwa mwishoni mwa yote, nitapata kuwa pamoja Naye anayenipenda zaidi. Uhusiano huu wa kina na imani yangu binafsi huniruhusu kuheshimu imani ya mtu mwingine bila kuhitaji kupuuza imani zangu au zao.

Katika kudumisha mipaka hii, naweza kupoteza wale watakaotafsiri vibaya kwa makusudi kwa sababu wana majeraha ambayo hayajaponya kuhusu suala la dini. Naweza kuonekana kama sisiheshimu imani ya mwingine kwa kuwa mwaminifu kwa yangu. Lakini maadamu sishtutumu, kulinganisha, au kuzungumza kwa ukatili kuhusu dini nyingine, najua kuwa ninajitendea uaminifu na pia ninawasimamia wengine. Sina shida kushtakiwa kwa uwongo kwani matendo yangu—kazi za ubunifu, maneno na sanaa—yanafunua mengi kuhusu asili yangu, hata wasipojua kwa nini moyo wangu unamtanguliza Mshonaji, hata wakati ni vigumu.

Sinaacha kuongea, kuimba au kushuhudia furaha ya Bwana katika maisha yangu. Ninachagua Upendo, kwa sababu niliumbwa kwa Upendo na Upendo Mwenyewe, kwa ajili ya Upendo. Jinsi Anavyotumia mimi kuwapa wale wanaohitaji zaidi daima itakuwa kwa njia nzuri zaidi kwa sababu itawafanya wengine wajue kwa nini Mwezeshaji ndiye aliye, na si mwingine yeyote.

Mipaka yako ya kiroho itakuwa yako.
Kwangu mimi, ndiyo sehemu muhimu zaidi ya mimi.

Yako ni yapi?

Psychological Boundaries

"The Lord is my Shepherd; I shall not want"

- Psalm 23 : 1

My psychological boundaries protect the unlearning process of my old patterns and are kind to those who interact with me during different seasons when I am transitioning into new ones.

In maintaining these boundaries, I might be coldly isolated, I might be looked down upon. I might be held in contempt. I do not mind this, not because I do not feel hurt, or sad or even abandoned, but because I know it is good to let the Weaver fill me with what no human can.

I have learned what my triggers are in this way. I have learned to meet them head on with compassion. I have learned to honour every fear, every need, and every want and allowed whatever comes up to surrender to the Lord who makes all things new in His time.

Your psychological boundaries will be different.
For me, they are the ones that teach us to grow.

What are yours?

Psikolojik Sınırlar

"Rab benim çobanımdır; hiçbir şeyim eksik olmaz."

- Mezmur 23:1

Psikolojik sınırlarım, eski kalıplarımı unutma sürecini korur ve yeni kalıplara geçiş yaptığım farklı dönemlerde benimle etkileşime girenlere karşı nazik davranır.

Bu sınırları korurken, soğuk bir şekilde izole edilebilirim, hor görülebilirim. Aşağılanabilirim. Bunu umursamıyorum, çünkü incinmiyorum, üzülmüyorum, hatta terk edilmiş hissetmiyorum, ama Dokumacının beni hiçbir insanın dolduramayacağı şeyle doldurmasına izin vermenin iyi olduğunu biliyorum.

Bu şekilde tetikleyicilerimin ne olduğunu öğrendim. Onlarla şefkatle yüzleşmeyi öğrendim. Her korkuyu, her ihtiyacı ve her isteği onurlandırmayı öğrendim ve ortaya çıkan her şeyi, her şeyi kendi zamanında yenileyen Rab'be teslim etmeyi öğrendim.

Sizin psikolojik sınırlarınız farklı olacaktır.
Benim için, bunlar bize büyümeyi öğreten sınırlardır.

Sizinkiler nelerdir?

Mipaka ya Kisaikolojia

"Bwana ndiye mchungaji wangu; sitaliwa na uhaba"

- Zaburi 23 : 1

Mipaka yangu ya kisaikolojia inalinda mchakato wa kuachana na tabia zangu za zamani na ni ya upole kwa wale wanaoshirikiana nami katika misimu tofauti ninapokuwa nikihamia kwenye mipya.

Katika kudumisha mipaka hii, naweza kujitenga kwa ukali, naweza kudharauliwa. Naweza kuchukiwa. Sijali kuhusu hili, si kwa sababu sihisi maumivu, au huzuni au hata kuachwa, bali kwa sababu najua ni vyema kumruhusu Mwezaji anijaze kile ambacho hakuna binadamu anayeweza.

Nimejifunza vichocheo vyangu kwa njia hii. Nimejifunza kuvikabili moja kwa moja kwa huruma. Nimejifunza kuheshimu kila hofu, kila hitaji, na kila tamaa na kuruhusu chochote kinachojitokeza kujisalimisha kwa Bwana anayefanya vitu vyote kuwa vipya kwa wakati Wake.

Mipaka yako ya kisaikolojia itakuwa tofauti.
Kwangu mimi, ni ile inayotufundisha kukua.

Yako ni yapi?

Mental Boundaries

"For I know the plans I have for you"

- Jeremiah 29 : 11

My mental boundaries protect the working space of my mind. It allows me to choose what feeds its beautiful journey, helps me recentre its direction when I accidentally wander and it honours the purpose of existence I have been given while also, making space to welcome others into it at the right time.

In maintaining these boundaries, I won't be easily tempted towards distractions. I might be doubted for choosing my creative path when they see no visible growth on the outside. I might be judged for not fulfilling others' expectations. I have accepted the consequences.

I am discovering my potential when I focus on what I need to do. I am uncovering my dreams in my heart ink when I structure the imagination of their shelves. I am working with whatever limitations and realizing their limitless possibilities.

Your mental boundaries will be unique.
For me, they are the ones that direct my purpose.

What are yours?

Zihinsel Sınırlar

"Çünkü sizin için yaptığım planları biliyorum."

- Yeremya 29:11

Zihinsel sınırlarım, zihnimin çalışma alanını korur. Bu sınırlar, zihnimin güzel yolculuğunu besleyen şeyleri seçmeme izin verir, yanlışlıkla yolumu kaybettiğimde yönümü yeniden bulmama yardımcı olur ve bana verilen varoluş amacını onurlandırırken, doğru zamanda başkalarını da bu alana kabul etmek için yer açar.

Bu sınırları koruyarak, dikkatimi dağıtan şeylere kolayca kapılmam. Dışarıdan görünür bir büyüme görmediklerinde, yaratıcı yolumu seçtiğim için şüpheyle karşılanabilirim. Başkalarının beklentilerini karşılamadığım için yargılanabilirim. Sonuçlarını kabul ettim.

Yapmam gerekenlere odaklandığımda potansiyelimi keşfediyorum. Hayallerimin raflarını yapılandırdığımda, kalbimdeki mürekkeple hayallerimi ortaya çıkarıyorum. Her türlü sınırlamayla çalışıyorum ve sınırsız olanaklarını fark ediyorum.

Zihinsel sınırlarınız benzersiz olacaktır.
Benim için, bunlar amacımı yönlendiren sınırlardır.

Sizinkiler nelerdir?

Mipaka ya Kifikra

"Kwa maana mimi najua mawazo ninayowawazia ninyi"

- Yeremia 29:11

Mipaka yangu ya kiakili inalinda eneo la kazi la akili yangu. Inaniruhusu kuchagua kile kinacholisha safari yake nzuri, inanisaidia kurekebisha mwelekeo wake ninapopotea kwa bahati mbaya na inaheshimu kusudi la uwepo nililopewa, huku pia, ikitengeneza nafasi ya kuwakaribisha wengine ndani yake kwa wakati unaofaa.

Katika kudumisha mipaka hii, sitavutiwa kwa urahisi na vishawishi vya kupoteza mwelekeo. Ninaweza kutilia shaka kwa kuchagua njia yangu ya ubunifu wanapoona hakuna ukuaji unaoonekana kwa nje. Ninaweza kuhukumiwa kwa kutotimiza matarajio ya wengine. Nimeyukubali matokeo yake.

Ninagundua uwezo wangu ninapozingatia kile ninachohitaji kufanya. Ninadhihirisha ndoto zangu katika wino wa moyo wangu ninapotengeneza muundo wa mawazo ya rafu zao. Ninatumia vikwazo vyovyote vilivyopo na kutambua uwezekano wake usio na kikomo.

Mipaka yako ya kiakili itakuwa ya kipekee.
Kwangu mimi, ndizo zinazoongoza kusudi langu.

Zako ni zipi?

Emotional Boundaries

"Hide me under the shadow of your wings."

- Psalm 17 : 8

My emotional boundaries protect my heart—its colourful petals of beauty, its wild waves of ocean, and its sensitive gravity of feeling everything in a big way, and yet it unveils its layers to those who take the time to truly understand it.

In maintaining these boundaries, I might be seen as stuck up or accused of being made of ice. I might be underestimated and made to feel invisible. I might be pressured to fall in line to fit in with what is known or popular. I have made my peace with being a misfit.

I can open my heart to let people in, but I can choose who I don't want to know me in there. This doesn't indicate that I don't care, think about or love the ones I keep at a distance. It just means I am conserving my energy for the things that matter because I am the one who has to be responsible for the feelings I have or allow when I share my inner world with others.

Your emotional boundaries will be layered.
For me, they are the ones that can hold my depths.

What are yours?

Duygusal Sınırlar

"Beni kanatlarının gölgesinde sakla."

- Mezmur 17:8

Duygusal sınırlarım kalbimi korur — onun renkli güzellikteki yaprakları, vahşi okyanus dalgaları ve her şeyi büyük bir şekilde hissetme konusundaki hassas çekim gücü. Yine de, onu gerçekten anlamak için zaman ayıranlara katmanlarını açığa çıkarır.

Bu sınırları korurken, kibirli olarak görülebilirim veya buz gibi olduğumla suçlanabilirim. Küçümsenebilir ve görünmez hissettirilebilirim. Bilinen veya popüler olan şeylere uymak için baskı görebilirim. Uyumsuz olmakla barıştım.

İnsanları içime almak için kalbimi açabilirim, ama orada beni tanımak istemediklerimi seçebilirim. Bu, uzak tuttuğum kişileri umursamadığım, düşünmediğim veya sevmediğim anlamına gelmez. Sadece, iç dünyamı başkalarıyla paylaştığımda hissettiğim veya izin verdiğim duygulardan sorumlu olan kişi ben olduğum için, önemli şeyler için enerjimi koruduğum anlamına gelir.

Duygusal sınırlarınız katmanlı olacaktır.
Benim için, bunlar benim derinliklerimi tutabilen sınırlardır.

Sizinkiler nelerdir?

Mipaka ya Kihisia

"Nifichie chini ya kivuli cha mabawa yako."

- Zaburi 17 : 8

Mipaka yangu ya kihisia inalinda moyo wangu—petali zake za rangi za uzuri, mawimbi yake ya porini ya bahari, na uzito wake mnyeti wa kuhisi kila kitu kwa kina, na bado huonyesha tabaka zake kwa wale wanaochukua muda kuelewa kwa kweli.

Katika kudumisha mipaka hii, naweza kuonekana kama mtu mwenye kiburi au kushtakiwa kuwa mtu mgumu. Naweza kudharauliwa na kufanywa nijihisi kama sisionekani. Naweza kushinikizwa kufuata mkondo ili kuendana na kile kinachojulikana au maarufu. Nimejipatanisha na hali ya kutofanana na wengine.

Naweza kufungua moyo wangu kuwaruhusu watu waingie, lakini naweza kuchagua ni nani sitakayemtaka anijue ndani yake. Hii haimaanishi kuwa sijali, sifikiri, au siwapendi wale ninaowaweka mbali. Inamaanisha tu ninahifadhi nguvu zangu kwa ajili ya mambo muhimu kwa sababu mimi ndiye anayehitaji kuwajibika kwa hisia ninazokuwa nazo au ninazoruhusu ninaposhiriki ulimwengu wangu wa ndani na wengine.

Mipaka yako ya kihisia itakuwa na tabaka.
Kwangu mimi, ndiyo inayoweza kuhifadhi kina changu.

Yako ni yapi?

Financial Boundaries

"...With the measure you use, it will be measured to you."

- Luke 6 : 38

My financial boundaries protect my well-being and others as well when I set limitations, usage, and expectations around money, assets, or other resources, depending on what season I am in.

In maintaining these boundaries, I might be resented or judged for saying "No" when I cannot and when I give generously. I might have love, affection, and kindness withdrawn for stating what I need. I might not be appreciated for upholding accountability when I lend money.

I can choose not to give anything I earn, regardless of what others presume, pressure, or project. I can receive help from an accountable partner to manage what is mine when dealing with bonds that don't respect my boundaries. I have the right to decide if, when, who, how, where, why and how much I want to give what I earn.

Your financial boundaries will be varied.
For me, they reveal who people are.

What are yours?

Mali Sınırlar

"...Kullandığınız ölçüyle, size de ölçülecektir."

- Luka 6:38

Mali sınırlarım, bulunduğum döneme bağlı olarak para, varlıklar veya diğer kaynaklar konusunda sınırlar, kullanım ve beklentiler belirlediğimde, benim ve başkalarının refahını korur.

Bu sınırları korurken, yapamadığım zaman "Hayır" dediğimde veya cömert davrandığımda kızılabilir veya yargılanabilirim. İhtiyacımı dile getirdiğim için sevgi, şefkat ve nezaketten mahrum kalabilirim. Borç verdiğimde sorumluluklarımı yerine getirdiğim için takdir edilmeyebilirim.

Başkalarının varsayımları, baskıları veya beklentileri ne olursa olsun, kazandıklarımı vermemeyi seçebilirim. Sınırlarımı saygı duymayan bağlarla uğraşırken, benim olanı yönetmek için sorumlu bir ortaktan yardım alabilirim. Kazandıklarımı vermek isteyip istemediğime, ne zaman, kime, nasıl, nerede, neden ve ne kadar vereceğime karar verme hakkına sahibim.

Finansal sınırlarınız farklılık gösterecektir.
Benim için, bu sınırlar insanların kim olduğunu ortaya çıkarır.
Sizinkiler nelerdir?

Mipaka ya Kifedha

"...Kwa kipimo mnachopima, ndivyo mtakapopimwa ninyi."

- Luka 6 : 38

Mipaka yangu ya kifedha inalinda ustawi wangu na pia wa wengine ninapoweka mipaka, matumizi, na matarajio kuhusu pesa, mali, au rasilimali nyingine, kulingana na hatua niliyonayo.

Katika kudumisha mipaka hii, naweza kuchukizwa au kuhukumiwa kwa kusema "Hapana" wakati siwezi na ninapotoa kwa ukarimu. Naweza kupokonywa upendo, huruma, na wema kwa kusema ninachohitaji. Naweza kutothaminiwa kwa kusimamia uwajibikaji ninapokopa pesa.

Ninaweza kuchagua kutoa chochote ninachopata, bila kujali kile wengine wanachodhania, kunishinikiza, au wanatarajia. Ninaweza kupokea msaada kutoka kwa mshirika anayewajibika ili kusimamia kile changu ninapokabiliana na uhusiano ambao hauheshimu mipaka yangu. Nina haki ya kuamua kama, lini, nani, vipi, wapi, kwa nini na kiasi gani ninataka kutoa ninachopata.

Mipaka yako ya kifedha itatofautiana.
Kwangu mimi, inadhihirisha watu walivyo.
Vyako ni vipi?

Physical Boundaries

"This is now bone of my bones and flesh of my flesh."

- Genesis 2 : 23

My physical boundaries define my personal space, what kind of intimate contact I allow and everything related to my health. They also give others a guideline on how to approach me without crossing them.

In maintaining these boundaries, I might feel anxiety because others might not understand or value. I might be judged by others' ego or misunderstandings or their own narratives when I don't give detailed reasons (except to my partner) about something that affects me deeply and that's okay. I might be looked at strangely for no longer being as tactile as I used to be.

I speak up when I feel my boundaries were violated. I no longer explain myself for not wanting to hug or be hugged by anyone who I feel has animosity or unspoken resentment towards me. I love being hugged, but only by those I love and who I know love me deeply without conditions. I love my body, beauty, and becoming even if others make negative comments in front or behind my back.

Your physical boundaries will be intuitive.
For me, they should be based on honesty.

What are yours?

Fiziksel Sınırlar

"Bu artık benim kemiklerimden ve etimden."

- Yaratılış 2:23

Fiziksel sınırlarım kişisel alanımı, ne tür samimi temaslara izin verdiğimi ve sağlığımla ilgili her şeyi tanımlar. Ayrıca başkalarına bu sınırları aşmadan bana nasıl yaklaşacakları konusunda bir kılavuz sağlar.

Bu sınırları korumak, başkalarının anlamaması veya değer vermemesi nedeniyle endişe hissetmeme neden olabilir. Beni derinden etkileyen bir şey hakkında (partnerim hariç) ayrıntılı nedenler vermediğimde, başkalarının egoları, yanlış anlamaları veya kendi anlatımları nedeniyle yargılanabilirim ve bu normaldir. Eskisi kadar dokunaklı olmadığım için tuhaf bakılabilirim.

Sınırlarımın ihlal edildiğini hissettiğimde sesimi çıkarırım. Bana karşı düşmanlık veya söylenmemiş bir kin beslediğini hissettiğim kimseyi kucaklamak veya kucaklanmak istemediğim için artık kendimi açıklamıyorum. Kucaklanmayı seviyorum, ama sadece sevdiğim ve beni koşulsuz olarak derinden sevdiğini bildiğim kişiler tarafından. Başkaları önümde veya arkamda olumsuz yorumlar yapsalar bile bedenimi, güzelliğimi ve kendimi seviyorum.

Fiziksel sınırlarınız sezgisel olacaktır.
Benim için bunlar dürüstlüğe dayanmalıdır.

Sizinkiler nelerdir?

Mipaka ya Kimwili

"Huyu sasa ni mfupa wa mifupa yangu

na nyama ya nyama zangu."

- Mwanzo 2:23

Mipaka yangu ya kimwili huainisha nafasi yangu binafsi, aina ya mgusano wa karibu ninaoruhusu na kila kitu kinachohusiana na afya yangu. Pia huwapa wengine mwongozo wa jinsi ya kunikaribia bila kuvuka mipaka hiyo.

Katika kudumisha mipaka hii, naweza kuhisi wasiwasi kwa sababu wengine wanaweza wasielewe au wasithamini. Naweza kuhukumiwa na ubinafsi wa wengine au kutoelewana au simulizi zao wenyewe ninapotoa sababu za kina (isipokuwa kwa mpenzi wangu) kuhusu jambo linalonigusa sana na hilo ni sawa. Naweza kutazamwa kwa ajabu kwa sababu sijali kugusana kama zamani.

Ninasema ninapohisi mipaka yangu imekiukwa. Sijali tena kujieleza kwa kutotaka kukumbatia au kukumbatiwa na yeyote ninayehisi ana chuki au kinyongo kisichosemwa dhidi yangu. Napenda kukumbatiwa, lakini ni na wale tu ninaowapenda na ninajua wanapenda kwa dhati bila masharti. Ninapenda mwili wangu, urembo wangu, na jinsi ninavyozidi kuwa mzuri hata kama wengine wanatoa maoni hasi mbele yangu au nyuma yangu.

Mipaka yako ya kimwili itakuwa ya hisia za ndani.
Kwangu mimi, inapaswa kuwa na msingi wa uaminifu.

Yako ni yapi?

Spatial Boundaries

"David danced before the Lord with all his might..."

- Samuel 6 : 14

My spatial boundaries protect my physical environment, personal property and creative places where I can take a break, flow, and just be wild. They also allow others to interact with me from these angles.

In maintaining these boundaries, I might be accused of being selfish because I am choosing a path that may or may not prosper. I might be treated like a burden, seen as unworthy and not important because people often treat you based on what worldly standards they think you should have to be significant to them. I might have to put up with less by accepting the bare minimum because not everyone wishes to support what they lacked the courage to do or even gracefully celebrate your wins, no matter which season they were in.

I have the right to keep my working space clean, unstructured or messy. I can choose what path I want to focus on every day. I am allowed to be happy doing what I was created to do, whether that is writing, painting, editing, collaborating, building, and dreaming.

Your space boundaries will be uneven.
For me, they are seasonal.

What are yours?

Mekansal Sınırlar

"Davut tüm gücüyle Rab'bin önünde dans etti..."

- Samuel 6 : 14

Mekansal sınırlarım, fiziksel çevrem, kişisel mülkiyetim ve dinlenebileceğim, akışına bırakabileceğim ve sadece kendim olabileceğim yaratıcı mekanlarımı korur. Ayrıca başkalarının da bu açılardan benimle etkileşime girmesine izin verir.

Bu sınırları korurken, başarılı olabilecek ya da olmayabilecek bir yol seçtiğim için bencil olmakla suçlanabilirim. İnsanlar genellikle size, kendileri için önemli olmanız gerektiğini düşündükleri dünyevi standartlara göre davrandıkları için, bir yük gibi muamele görebilir, değersiz ve önemsiz olarak görülebilirim. Herkes, cesaret edemediği şeyleri desteklemek veya hangi dönemde olursa olsun, başarılarınızı nezaketle kutlamak istemeyebileceğinden, asgari düzeyde kabul ederek daha azıyla yetinmek zorunda kalabilirim.

Çalışma alanımı temiz, düzensiz veya dağınık tutma hakkım var. Her gün hangi yola odaklanmak istediğimi seçebilirim. Yazmak, resim yapmak, düzenlemek, işbirliği yapmak, inşa etmek ve hayal kurmak gibi, yaratıldığım şeyi yaparken mutlu olmaya hakkım var.

Alan sınırlarınız düzensiz olacaktır.
Benim için bunlar mevsimseldir.

Sizinkiler nedir?

Mipaka ya Nafasi

"Daudi akacheza mbele za Bwana kwa nguvu zake zote..."

- Samweli 6 : 14

Mipaka yangu ya nafasi inalinda mazingira yangu ya kimwili, mali yangu binafsi na maeneo yangu ya ubunifu ambapo naweza kupumzika, kujieleza, na kuwa mchangamfu tu. Pia inawaruhusu wengine kuingiliana nami kutoka kwa mitazamo hii.

Katika kudumisha mipaka hii, naweza kushtakiwa kwa ubinafsi kwa sababu ninachagua njia ambayo inaweza kufanikiwa au la. Ninaweza kutendewa kama mzigo, kuonekana si wa maana na asiye muhimu kwa sababu mara nyingi watu wanakutendea kulingana na viwango vya kidunia wanavyofikiri unapaswa kuwa navyo ili uwe na maana kwao. Huenda nikalazimika kuvumilia kidogo kwa kukubali kile cha chini kabisa kwa sababu si kila mtu anataka kuunga mkono kile ambacho hakukuwa na ujasiri wa kukifanya au hata kusherehekea kwa unyenyekevu ushindi wako, bila kujali walikuwa katika msimu gani.

Nina haki ya kuweka nafasi yangu ya kazi ikiwa safi, isiyo na mpangilio au yenye fujo. Naweza kuchagua njia ninayotaka kuijikita kila siku. Ninaruhusiwa kuwa na furaha nikifanya kile nilichoundwa kufanya, iwe ni kuandika, kupaka rangi, kuhariri, kushirikiana, kujenga, na kuota ndoto.

Mipaka yako ya nafasi haitakuwa sawa.
Kwangu mimi, ni ya misimu.

Yako ni yapi?

Space For You

Self-Boundaries For You

Space For You

Reena Doss

The Lanterns

Space For You

∞

Acknowledgements

I am grateful

Boundaries are important internal and external edges that are necessary to uphold, especially when you know the truth of who you are. If you understand the attributes you value most, you will know how to shape, form, and create personal boundaries—whether spiritual, psychological, mental, emotional, financial, physical, or spatial.

When boundaries are centred around these categories, accepting what feeds your soul—and withdrawing from situations that diminish who you are—becomes easier. This acceptance is not often realized as self-affirmations becoming clearer, yet it allows one to be mentally healthy, feel good about their own well-being, and also hold their own peace.

Most people want peace without discovering what kind of peace they are looking to cultivate. Often, it is about identifying one's truth in regard to attributes, boundaries, and affirmations, and giving yourself permission to claim them as your right. Maintaining this right may disrupt your life into seeming chaos, because not everyone you love—or who says they love you—will respect it.

You may lose the ones you love: people, things, and even your comfort. They may say you changed. This is true. You have, and that's okay. They remember an old version of you that no longer exists—the one that was easier to manipulate, walk over, and who chose themselves over you. And who they still are will want to keep you in a place they comprehend, choosing to see you in the way they want and dismissing where you've grown.

Many (not all) will take advantage of what you share, especially if they have access to you and those close to you. When they think your growth depends on their approval or validation, that is a clear sign of a toxic connection. Remember this. Forget inconsistent words or breadcrumbed love that showed up when, in truth, giving was being measured through the lens of conditional love by people who had forgotten how to be unconditional.

Don't doubt what was revealed in silence, especially when your value was being hidden.

You don't have to cut those who haven't grown with you. Wait for them. You don't have to be angry with those who cannot meet you where you have walked through. Help them kindly. You don't have to feel guilty about distancing yourself from those who sabotaged you behind your back yet gave you false words of solidarity, simply because they gifted you what was only easy to them but mattered a great deal to you. Wish them well. This does not mean you must lessen, dishonour, or undervalue what they brought to your life. But do not forget what you brought to theirs as well, even when it cost you personal sacrifice, comfort, and tears that they may not know about. Recognise your worth, allow yourself to receive and meet those who know your worth too.

Some will not want to share your load when it is inconvenient to their comfort. In fact, they will see your hard times as a hinderance to where they are already at ease, not because they are bad but because they are weak-willed and not willing to understand the struggles you are going through or have conquered. They are unaware of their own gaps, fears, and shadows and are not willing to face them.

A few will distance themselves because they would rather see where you lack than where they are. Know the difference between those who walked into the fire with you and those who made excuses not to. The latter know they will lose familiarity, so they would rather see you as the cause of their problems instead of appreciating your resilience—to heal from trauma, rebuild from nothing, and restore the parts of you that broke down while they witnessed it—but secretly blamed you for whatever befell you, and even stood by those who contributed to your pain, despite your speaking up about it.

You know the ones who preferred you when you were struggling, and you will see this in how they support your growth—some will do it half-heartedly, others will make excuses, and many will publicly pretend to be there for you only when it feels like where you are headed is a sure thing for them to be seen. This is human nature, but it is not going to add to your peace.

∞

For some reason, these very same people will suddenly take credit for your glow as if it belongs to them, simply because you honoured their presence in whatever you did.

The truth is... they chose to become witnesses to your journey, unlike the ones who were direct participants in everything. Both—the spectator observer and the gladiator warrior type—should not become intertwined with who you are becoming, no matter how long they have been in your life. This is because, when you are being obedient to a purpose given to you, you must allow only the Weaver to define who you are.

This becomes a blessing to the gladiator warriors when your light is brightest, and a hard boundary to the spectator observers who abandoned you when the night was darkest. Some dance in between, but those are the most dangerous to trust. This is because they reveal where their true loyalty lies—it is dependent on who you are connected to, rather than on you.

Gladiator warriors are the ones who leave your side to tend to things that matter only when they know you are no longer wounded or broken. Spectator observers, on the other hand, will call you toxic, say you are draining, and judge you, especially when they should have been there the most.

Over time, with the right boundaries, practicing affirmations, and being honest about where you are in terms of what you value, you learn who to trust. You observe who is in your corner. You discover who showed up consistently—not just watched you. You notice those who support you no matter what you do, even if it wasn't obvious right away. But you also learn there are many who will only study you to see what they can get, not what they can give or how they can support you.

This is why it is important to be bold, truthful, and confident about where you stand on faith, principles, attributes, purpose, roots, choices, and causes.

I am so thankful to everyone—no matter how small or big, peaceful or chaotic, loyal or disloyal—especially to *Ink Gladiators Press' team: Leonie Belle Hawk,* who taught me to see the finer details in the bigger picture, even when I have not always wanted to believe what I saw, especially when it was staring straight at me*; Justin Adam Wolf* and *Aelius Arche,* my editorial team, for working diligently on editing and proofing because it let me wear other hats that I needed to complete my work.

I want to thank the ones who truly invested in my peace, stayed consistently close to my journey, and believed in my voices from the very beginning. I especially want to thank many people for their words and actions, which only served as reminders that helped me discern alignment with my journey of dreams, creativity, and love for writing. I would like to think a few in the community supported my work when they could, as well as encouraged self-worth in themselves and others. I have always enjoyed deep discussions about many things with a few, though our schedules never seemed to meet, which made me see that that too was redirection towards my purpose.

When the Weaver strips you of everything, it is always the truth that remains. And that truth is the most precious pearl of all, because it is wrapped in a peace that is neither taken, borrowed, nor dependent on anyone else.

I am grateful.

May the quill of hope find you in the dark,

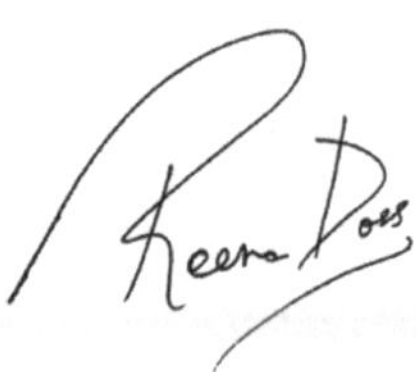

Reena Doss

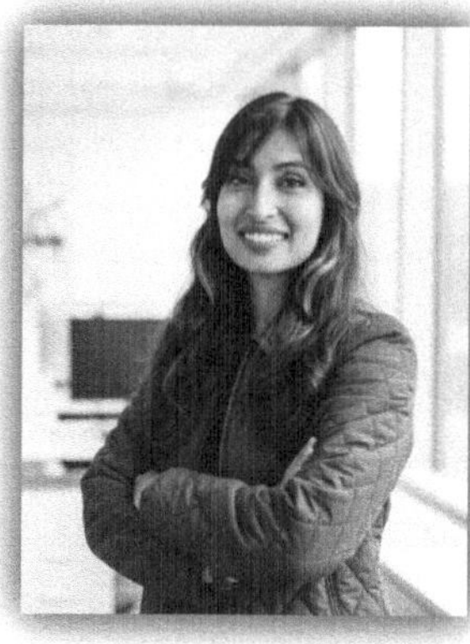

I'll find you in the dark...

Born in Calcutta with roots drawn from Chennai and Pondicherry, Reena Doss has lived most of her life in the south of India—Bangalore. Though she prefers traveling to far-off places inside her head, she sometimes ventures into the world that others call real.

Reena Doss considers writing to be her first voice of expression, followed closely by art, and creativity. Through the encouraging platform provided by the Instagram community, she reclaimed her lost voices, evolved a few others and discovered new ones along the way.

This has redeemed her trust that consistent Hope, Faith and Love in what is true ignites what is impossible to occur. Her adoration for her beloved Weaver, the Celestial Sky, Nature and her fellow Earthians has given her immeasurable courage to endure every season with a resilience born from battles overcome.

You can try and catch her but it may not always be possible as she is generally off on adventures flying on phoenix wings, swimming into the deep with mermaids and chasing fiery dragons down for stories.

To those who remain true to themselves,
to those who create magic wherever they go,
and for those who sit beside the hurt
when everyone else leaves,
Art will always immortalize you.

Please scan the QR code to follow her on
Instagram @reenadossauthor
www.reenadoss.com

This little book is called a *Lantern* because love is light in disguise. It can only be found when you are buried in the dark, when the seeds die, and you choose to bravely grow and become worthy of your given name—a polished gem, a diamond that cannot help but shine. Lanterns are meant for those who need hope while they are being:

- ♥ Condemned unjustly by those who see a version they want
- ♥ Gossiped about when they are not present to defend themselves
- ♥ Taken advantage of when they were beaten down by life, by those who should have stood by them
- ♥ Judged, neglected, and persecuted while they are struggling
- ♥ Abandoned by those who willingly chose to see them as toxic because it suited their narrative
- ♥ Manipulated by those who bore false witness against them to take what wasn't theirs
- ♥ Gaslit, broken, and their truth erased while they were at their most vulnerable
- ♥ Hated, harassed, and purposefully pressured into giving up on who they are because of others' jealousy
- ♥ Trying to process trauma to speak in a language that isn't being heard
- ♥ Eagerly isolated by loved ones on the advice of others who can't understand them any more
- ♥ Neglected by those whose promises dimmed when things got difficult
- ♥ Treated as outcasts by those who expect their will to be done
- ♥ Mocked for what they do just because it is different and does not fit into any box

Promoting hope and unwrapping the stigma of mental health

For any inquiries, please email us at contact@inkgladiatorspress.com.

Please scan the QR Code below if you would like to follow us

on Instagram @inkgladiatorspress.

Ink Gladiators Press®

Publishing and promoting warriors on life's battlefield

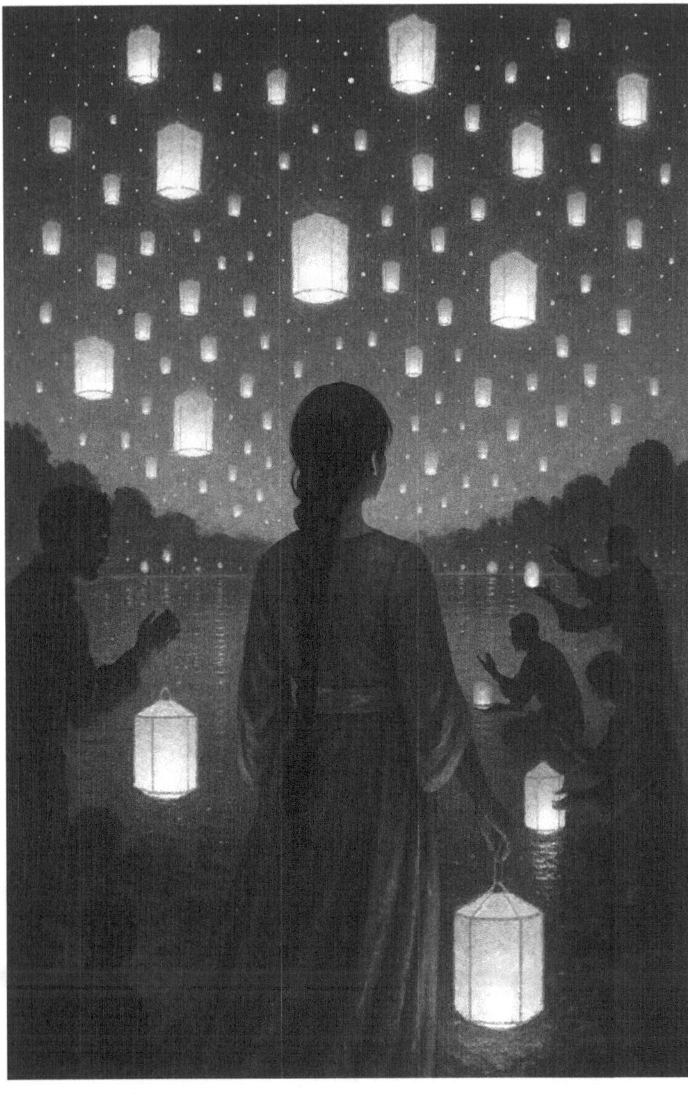

Printed at Repro India Ltd.